Low Sodium Tasty Recipes

Tasty and Incredibly Healthy Low Sodium Meals to Enjoy Your Diet and Lose Weight

Jennifer Loyel

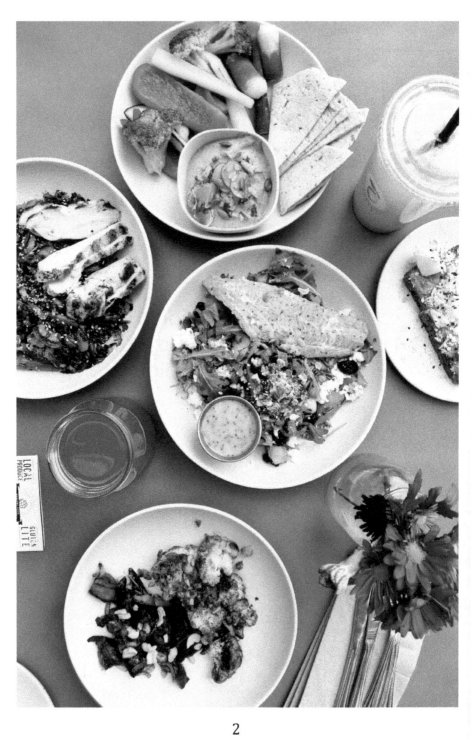

professional advice. The content within this book has been derived from various sources. Please consult a licensed professional before attempting any techniques outlined in this book.

By reading this document, the reader agrees that under no circumstances is the author responsible for any losses, direct or indirect, which are incurred as a result of the use of information contained within this document, including, but not limited to, — errors, omissions, or inaccuracies.

Table of Contents

French Glazed Green Beans

Servings: 4

Ingredients:

- 1/4 cup chopped walnuts
- 4 teaspoons cold-pressed walnut or canola oil
- 2 (15-ounce) cans French-cut green beans
- 1 teaspoon lemon juice
- 1 teaspoon honey
- 1 teaspoon French Spice Blend
- 1/8 teaspoon grated lemon zest
- 1/8 teaspoon mustard powder
- 1/8 teaspoon freshly ground black pepper

Directions:

1. Bring a large, deep nonstick sauté pan to temperature over medium heat. Add the walnuts. Toast for 3 minutes, stirring frequently so the walnuts don't burn. Transfer to a bowl and set aside.

2. Add the walnut or canola oil to the pan. Drain the green beans and add to the pan; stir to toss in the oil. Once the green beans are hot, push them to the sides of the pan.

3. In a medium bowl, add the lemon juice, honey, French spice blend, lemon zest, mustard powder, and pepper; stir to combine. Toss the green beans in the lemon juice mixture. Pour into a serving bowl and top with the toasted walnuts.

Nutrition Info: (Per Serving):Calories: 88; Total Fat: 5 g; Saturated Fat: 0 g; Cholesterol: 0 mg; Protein: 1 g; Sodium: 29 mg; Potassium: 205 mg; Fiber: 3 g; Carbohydrates: 9 g; Sugar: 1 g

Tomato Gravy

Servings: 4

Ingredients:

- ¼ cup (40 g) onion, chopped
- 2 tablespoons (28 ml) vegetable oil
- 2 tablespoons (16 g) all-purpose flour
- 2 cups (360 g) tomatoes, chopped
- 1 cup (235 ml) skim milk
- ¼ teaspoon black pepper

Directions:

1. Sauté onion in oil. Stir in flour and brown. Add tomatoes, with juice; stir as gravy thickens. Add milk, a little at a time, and pepper, and cook until gravy is of desired thickness.

Nutrition Info: (Per Serving): 135 g water; 118 calories (53% from fat, 12% from protein, 35% from carb); 4 g protein; 7 g total fat; 1 g saturated fat; 2 g monounsaturated fat; 4 g polyunsaturated fat; 10 g carb; 1 g fiber; 2 g sugar; 99 mg calcium; 0 mg iron; 40 mg sodium; 309 mg potassium; 746 IU vitamin A; 11 mg vitamin C; 1 mg cholesterol

Creamy Mushroom Sauce

Servings: 4

Ingredients:

- 2 cups (140 g) mushrooms, sliced
- 1 onion, chopped
- 1 tablespoon (14 g) unsalted butter
- 4 ounces (115 g) cream cheese
- 2 tablespoons (16 g) all-purpose flour
- ¼ teaspoon white pepper
- 1 cup (235 ml) skim milk

Directions:

1. Sauté mushrooms and onion in the butter until tender. Stir in cream cheese until melted. Shake flour, pepper, and milk together. Add to skillet. Cook and stir until thickened and bubbly.

Nutrition Info: (Per Serving): 131 g water; 185 calories (62% from fat, 14% from protein, 24% from carb); 6 g protein; 13 g total fat; 8 g saturated fat; 4 g monounsaturated fat; 1 g polyunsaturated fat; 11 g carb; 1 g fiber; 2 g sugar; 120 mg calcium; 1 mg iron; 123 mg sodium; 305 mg potassium; 596 IU vitamin A; 3 mg vitamin C; 40 mg cholesterol

Sweet Potatoes, Squash, And Apples

Servings: 6

Ingredients:

- 2 cups (220 g) sweet potatoes, cut into 1-inch (2.5-cm) cubes
- 2 cups (450 g) butternut squash, cut into 1-inch (2.5-cm) cubes
- 1 apple, peeled and sliced
- ¼ cup (71 g) apple juice concentrate
- ½ teaspoon ground cinnamon

Directions:

1. Cook sweet potatoes and squash in water until almost soft. Drain and return to pan. Add apple and juice concentrate. Cook until apple is tender. Sprinkle with cinnamon.

Nutrition Info: (Per Serving): 149 g water; 122 calories (2% from fat, 6% from protein, 92% from carb); 2 g protein; 0 g total fat; 0 g saturated fat; 0 g monounsaturated fat; 0 g polyunsaturated fat; 30 g carb; 4 g fiber; 9 g sugar; 56 mg calcium; 1 mg iron; 33 mg sodium; 456 mg potassium; 9 IU vitamin A; 29 mg vitamin C; 0 mg cholesterol

Roasted Beets

Servings: 2

Ingredients:

- 2 beets, well-scrubbed but not peeled
- 1 teaspoon olive oil
- 1 teaspoon dried thyme

Directions:

1. Preheat the oven to 450°F (230°C, gas mark 8). Cut off the tops and root ends of the beets, then slice as thinly as possible (aim for about 1/8 inch [0.32 cm]). In a medium bowl, toss the beet slices with the olive oil, then add a sprinkling of thyme. Place beets in a single layer on 1 or 2 baking sheets and roast in a preheated oven for 20 to 25 minutes. Remove from the oven and allow to cool slightly.

Nutrition Info: (Per Serving): 72 g water; 57 calories (36% from fat, 9% from protein, 54% from carb); 1 g protein; 2 g total fat; 0 g saturated fat; 2 g monounsaturated fat; 0 g polyunsaturated fat; 8 g carb; 2 g fiber; 6 g sugar; 23 mg calcium; 1 mg iron; 64 mg sodium; 271 mg potassium; 46 IU vitamin A; 4 mg vitamin C; 0 mg cholesterol

Swiss Corn Bake

Servings: 6

Ingredients:

- 16 ounces (455 g) frozen corn
- 6 ounces (175 ml) evaporated skim milk
- 3 ounces (85 g) Swiss cheese, shredded, divided
- 2 eggs
- 2 tablespoons (20 g) onion, minced
- 1 cup (115 g) low sodium bread crumbs

Directions:

1. Combine corn, milk, about ¾ of the cheese, eggs, and onion. Place in a 10 × 6-inch (25 × 15-cm) greased baking dish. Combine bread crumbs with remaining cheese. Sprinkle on top. Bake at 350°F (180°C, gas mark 4) for 25 to 30 minutes.

Nutrition Info: (Per Serving): 96 g water; 197 calories (15% from fat, 18% from protein, 66% from carb); 9 g protein; 4 g total fat; 1 g saturated fat; 1 g monounsaturated fat; 1 g polyunsaturated fat; 34 g carb; 3 g fiber; 7 g sugar; 129 mg calcium; 2 mg iron;

70 mg sodium; 382 mg potassium; 390 IU vitamin A; 6 mg vitamin C; 83 mg cholesterol

Sweet Potato Mash

Servings: 4

Ingredients:

- 4 medium-size sweet potatoes, peeled and cubed
- 2 teaspoons lemon juice
- 4 teaspoons unsalted butter
- 1/4 teaspoon ground cumin
- 1/4 teaspoon ground cinnamon
- 1/4 teaspoon dried ginger
- Optional: 1/4 teaspoon chipotle powder or other salt-free chili powder
- 1/2 cup skim milk

Directions:

1. Put the sweet potatoes in a saucepan and cover with cold water. Add the lemon juice. Bring to a boil over medium heat. Cover and cook for 7–10 minutes, until the potatoes are fork tender. Once the sweet potatoes are fully cooked, drain the water from the pot and place them in a medium-size bowl.
2. Melt the butter in the saucepan over medium heat. Add the cumin, cinnamon, ginger, and

chipotle powder, if using; sauté the spices for 30 seconds. Add the milk and bring to a boil. Pour over the cooked sweet potatoes. Mix together using a masher or wooden spoon. Serve immediately.

Nutrition Info: (Per Serving):Calories: 161; Total Fat: 4 g; Saturated Fat: 2 g; Cholesterol: 10 mg; Protein: 3 g; Sodium: 57 mg; Potassium: 409 mg; Fiber: 3 g; Carbohydrates: 28 g; Sugar: 10 g

Baked Beans

Servings: 6

Ingredients:

- ½ pound (225 g) navy beans
- 4 cups (940 ml) water
- 1 cup (240 g) Chili Sauce
- ¾ cup (120 g) onion, chopped
- 2 tablespoons (40 g) molasses
- 2 tablespoons (30 g) brown sugar
- 1 ½ teaspoons dry mustard
- ¼ teaspoon garlic powder
- 1 cup (235 ml) water

Directions:

1. Place beans in water in large saucepan. Bring to a boil and cook for 1 minute. Remove from the heat and let stand for 1 hour. Return to heat and simmer until almost done, about 1 hour. Drain. Mix with remaining ingredients. Place in a 1 ½-quart (1 ½-L) baking dish. Cover and bake for 4 hours. Add water if needed during cooking.

Nutrition Info: (Per Serving): 253 g water; 65 calories (4% from fat, 5% from protein, 91% from carb); 1 g protein; 0 g total fat; 0 g saturated fat; 0 g monounsaturated fat; 0 g polyunsaturated fat; 15 g carb; 1 g fiber; 12 g sugar; 36 mg calcium; 1 mg iron; 17 mg sodium; 151 mg potassium; 670 IU vitamin A; 9 mg vitamin C; 0 mg cholesterol

Black Rice Pilaf

Servings: 6

Ingredients:

- 2 tablespoons unsalted butter
- 1 tablespoon olive oil
- 3 cloves garlic, sliced
- 1/2 cup sliced green onions
- 1 teaspoon grated lemon zest
- 11/2 cups black rice
- 3 cups Chicken Stock
- 1/8 teaspoon pepper
- 2 teaspoons minced fresh thyme leaves

Directions:

1. In heavy saucepan, melt butter with olive oil over medium-low heat. Add garlic and green onions; sauté for 2 minutes.
2. Add lemon zest and black rice; sauté for another 2–4 minutes, stirring constantly, until rice is slightly toasted.
3. Add stock and pepper and bring to a simmer. Reduce heat to low, cover the pan, and simmer for 30 minutes or until the rice is just tender.

4.   Remove pan from heat, stir in thyme, and let stand, covered, for 5 minutes. Fluff rice with a fork and serve.

Nutrition Info: (Per Serving):Calories: 241; Total Fat: 8 g; Saturated Fat: 3 g; Cholesterol: 10 mg; Protein: 6 g; Sodium: 38 mg; Potassium: 248 mg; Fiber: 3 g; Carbohydrates: 36 g; Sugar: 0 g

Veggie Hash

Servings: 6

Ingredients:

- 2 potatoes, shredded
- ½ cup (80 g) onion, shredded
- ¼ cup (30 g) red bell pepper, shredded
- ¼ cup (30 g) green bell pepper, shredded
- ¼ cup zucchini, shredded
- 2 tablespoons (28 ml) olive oil
- ⅓ cup (60 g) tomatoes, finely chopped

Directions:

1. Mix together all vegetables except tomatoes. Heat oil In a large skillet. Add vegetables and spread to an even layer. Cook until lightly browned. Turn over and add chopped tomatoes on top. Cover and cook until tender. Cut in wedges to serve.

Nutrition Info: (Per Serving): 108 g water; 135 calories (30% from fat, 6% from protein, 64% from carb); 2 g protein; 5 g total fat; 1 g saturated fat; 3 g monounsaturated fat; 1 g polyunsaturated fat; 22 g carb; 2 g fiber; 2 g sugar; 13 mg calcium; 0 mg iron; 7

mg sodium; 392 mg potassium; 190 IU vitamin A; 18 mg vitamin C; 0 mg cholesterol

Carrots With An English Accent

Servings: 4

Ingredients:

- Olive oil spray
- 1/4 cup water
- 1 teaspoon lemon juice
- 4 cups baby carrots, sliced
- 1 teaspoon English Spice Blend

Directions:

1. Preheat oven to 350°F.
2. Spray an ovenproof casserole dish with the olive oil spray. Add the water and lemon juice, and stir to combine.
3. Spread the carrot slices over the water-lemon mixture. Mist the carrots with the olive oil spray. Sprinkle the English spice blend over the carrots. Cover and bake for 35 minutes.
4. Mist the carrots again with the olive oil spray, if desired. Uncover and bake for an additional 10 minutes or until the carrots are tender.

Nutrition Info: (Per Serving):Calories: 50; Total Fat: 0 g; Saturated Fat: 0 g; Cholesterol: 0 mg; Protein: 1 g;

Sodium: 84 mg; Potassium: 391 mg; Fiber: 3 g; Carbohydrates: 11 g; Sugar: 5 g

Roasted Italian Vegetables

Servings: 2

Ingredients:

- 2 tablespoons (28 ml) olive oil
- 1 clove garlic, minced
- ½ teaspoon dried basil
- ½ teaspoon dried oregano
- ½ onion, sliced into wedges
- ½ green bell pepper, cut into 1-inch (2.5-cm) pieces
- ½ cup (90 g) plum tomatoes, split in half
- 1 cup zucchini, cut in 1-inch (2.5-cm) slices
- 4 ounces (115 g) mushrooms, cut in half
- Nonstick vegetable oil spray

Directions:

1. Combine oil, garlic, basil, and oregano in a resealable plastic bag. Add vegetables and shake to coat evenly. Spray a 9 × 13-inch (23 × 33-cm) roasting pan with cooking spray. Place the vegetables in a single layer in the pan. Roast at 400°F (200°C, gas mark 6) until crisp cooked, about 20 minutes.

Nutrition Info: (Per Serving): 209 g water; 172 calories (68% from fat, 8% from protein, 24% from carb); 4 g protein; 14 g total fat; 2 g saturated fat; 10 g monounsaturated fat; 2 g polyunsaturated fat; 11 g carb; 3 g fiber; 5 g sugar; 35 mg calcium; 1 mg iron; 13 mg sodium; 554 mg potassium; 606 IU vitamin A; 49 mg vitamin C; 0 mg cholesterol

Marinated Carrots

Servings: 6

Ingredients:

- 2 cups (260 g) carrots
- ¾ cup (150 g) sugar
- ¾ cup (175 ml) vinegar
- ¾ cup (175 ml) water
- 1 tablespoon (11 g) mustard seed
- 1 stick cinnamon
- 3 whole cloves

Directions:

1. Boil carrots for 5 minutes. Drain and cut into 3-inch (7.5-cm) sticks. Combine remaining ingredients and bring to a boil. Simmer for 10 minutes. Pour over carrots, cover, and refrigerate overnight. Drain and serve.

Nutrition Info: (Per Serving): 96 g water; 128 calories (4% from fat, 3% from protein, 93% from carb); 1 g protein; 1 g total fat; 0 g saturated fat; 0 g monounsaturated fat; 0 g polyunsaturated fat; 32 g carb; 2 g fiber; 29 g sugar; 26 mg calcium; 0 mg iron; 30 mg sodium; 180 mg potassium; 5137 IU vitamin A; 3 mg vitamin C; 0 mg cholesterol

Grilled Corn Succotash

Servings: 4

Ingredients:

- 4 ears Grilled Corn
- 1 (16-ounce) package frozen lima beans
- 2 tablespoons unsalted butter
- 1 medium onion, chopped
- 3 cloves garlic, minced
- 1 tablespoon grated fresh ginger root
- 1/4 teaspoon white pepper
- 2 tablespoons honey

Directions:

1. Cut the kernels off the cob and set aside. Thaw lima beans according to package directions and drain well.
2. In skillet, melt butter over medium heat. Add onion; cook and stir for 5 minutes or until crisp-tender.
3. Add garlic and ginger root; cook for another 1 minute or until fragrant. Add the corn, beans, pepper, and honey and bring to a simmer.

4. Simmer mixture for 5–6 minutes or until vegetables are tender, stirring frequently. Serve immediately.

Nutrition Info: (Per Serving):Calories: 266; Total Fat: 6 g; Saturated Fat: 3 g; Cholesterol: 15 mg; Protein: 9 g; Sodium: 37 mg; Potassium: 657 mg; Fiber: 8 g; Carbohydrates: 46 g; Sugar: 12 g

Mashed Sweet Potatoes With Caramelized Onions

Servings: 6

Ingredients:

- 4 large sweet potatoes
- 3 tablespoons unsalted butter
- 1/3 cup whole milk
- 1/4 cup heavy cream
- 2 tablespoons orange juice
- 2 tablespoons maple syrup
- 1 cup Slow Cooker Caramelized Onions
- 1 teaspoon dried thyme leaves
- 1/4 teaspoon white pepper

Directions:

1. Preheat oven to 375°F. Scrub the sweet potatoes and prick them with a fork. Place on a baking pan and bake for 55–65 minutes or until they are very tender.

2. Cool the potatoes for 20 minutes, then cut in half lengthwise and scoop out the flesh with a spoon into a large bowl. Add the butter and mash.

3. Stir in the milk, cream, orange juice, maple syrup, onions, thyme, and pepper. Pile into a 3-quart baking dish. Bake for 25–35 minutes or until hot and slightly brown on top.

Nutrition Info: (Per Serving):Calories: 203; Total Fat: 12 g; Saturated Fat: 6 g; Cholesterol: 29 mg; Protein: 2 g; Sodium: 25 mg; Potassium: 353 mg; Fiber: 2 g; Carbohydrates: 21 g; Sugar: 10 g

Grilled Mushroom And Vegetable Medley

Servings: 4

Ingredients:

- Olive oil spray
- 1 large red bell pepper, seeded
- 1 large green bell pepper, seeded
- 2 medium zucchini
- 2 medium yellow squashes
- 2 cups fresh button mushrooms
- 4 medium green onions, white and green parts minced
- 1 teaspoon dried thyme
- 1 teaspoon dried basil
- 1/2 teaspoon garlic powder
- 1/4 teaspoon mustard powder
- 1/8 teaspoon freshly ground black pepper
- Optional: Vinaigrette dressing of choice

Directions:

1. Prepare a 20" × 14" sheet of heavy-duty foil by spraying the center with the olive oil spray.
2. Cut the bell peppers into 1/4" strips; slice the zucchini and squashes crosswise into 1/4"

slices. Slice the mushrooms. Arrange the vegetables over the foil. Evenly sprinkle the green onions, thyme, basil, garlic powder, mustard powder, and black pepper over the vegetables. Lightly spray the mixture with the spray oil. Fold the ends of the foil up and over the vegetables, creating a packet and sealing it by crimping the edges well, leaving space for heat to circulate.

3.   Grill on a covered grill over medium coals for 20–25 minutes, or until the vegetables are fork tender. Carefully open the foil packet and grill for an additional 5 minutes to let the juices from the vegetables evaporate, if desired.

Nutrition Info: (Per Serving):Calories: 50; Total Fat: 0 g; Saturated Fat: 0 g; Cholesterol: 0 mg; Protein: 3 g; Sodium: 7 mg; Potassium: 569 mg; Fiber: 3 g; Carbohydrates: 10 g; Sugar: 5 g

Sweet Potato-peach Bake

Servings: 4

Ingredients:

- 1 pound (455 g) sweet potatoes
- 2 cups (400 g) peaches, drained and sliced
- ¼ cup (60 g) brown sugar
- ¼ cup (40g) cashews, unsalted
- ¼ teaspoon ground ginger

Directions:

1. Peel and slice the sweet potatoes and boil until almost done. Combine with peaches and place in an 8 × 8-inch (20 × 20-cm) baking dish. Combine the remaining ingredients and sprinkle over top. Bake at 350°F (180°C, gas mark 4) for 30 minutes.

Nutrition Info: (Per Serving): 201 g water; 240 calories (14% from fat, 6% from protein, 80% from carb); 4 g protein; 4 g total fat; 1 g saturated fat; 2 g monounsaturated fat; 1 g polyunsaturated fat; 50 g carb; 5 g fiber; 33 g sugar; 53 mg calcium; 2 mg iron; 42 mg sodium; 520 mg potassium; 476 IU vitamin A; 19 mg vitamin C; 0 mg cholesterol

Sweet And Sour Red Cabbage

Servings: 6

Ingredients:

- 4 cups (280 g) red cabbage, shredded
- 1 onion, chopped
- 1 apple, peeled and chopped
- ½ cup (115 g) brown sugar
- ½ cup (120 ml) cider vinegar

Directions:

1. Place vegetables in a slow cooker. Combine sugar and vinegar, pour over vegetables, and stir to mix. Cook on low for 7 to 8 hours.

Nutrition Info: (Per Serving): 109 g water; 109 calories (1% from fat, 4% from protein, 95% from carb); 1 g protein; 0 g total fat; 0 g saturated fat; 0 g monounsaturated fat; 0 g polyunsaturated fat; 28 g carb; 2 g fiber; 24 g sugar; 49 mg calcium; 1 mg iron; 24 mg sodium; 276 mg potassium; 671 IU vitamin A; 36 mg vitamin C; 0 mg cholesterol

Oven-roasted Corn On The Cob

Servings: 4

Ingredients:

- 4 ears fresh sweet corn
- 4 teaspoons fresh lime juice
- Freshly ground black pepper

Directions:

1. Preheat oven to 350°F.
2. Peel back the husks of the corn. Remove any silk. Brush the corn with the lime juice and generously grind black pepper over the corn. Pull the husks back up over the corn, twisting the husks at the top to keep them sealed over each ear.
3. Place the corn on the rack in a roasting pan large enough to hold the ears without overlapping. Roast for 30 minutes or until the corn is heated through and tender. Peel back the husks and use them as a handle, if desired, or discard the husks and insert corn holders into the ends of the cobs. Serve immediately.

Nutrition Info: (Per Serving):Calories: 60; Total Fat: 0 g; Saturated Fat: 0 g; Cholesterol: 0 mg; Protein: 2 g; Sodium: 2 mg; Potassium: 163 mg; Fiber: 1 g; Carbohydrates: 14 g; Sugar: 0 g

Orange Burgundy Chicken

Servings: 4

Ingredients:

- ¼ cup (75 g) orange marmalade
- ½ tablespoon cornstarch
- ¼ cup (60 ml) burgundy wine
- 4 boneless chicken breasts

Directions:

1. In a small saucepan, Combine the first 3 ingredients. Cook and stir until thickened and bubbly. Grill chicken breasts until done, about 15 minutes on a charcoal or gas grill (may also be baked in the oven). Brush sauce over chicken during last 5 minutes of cooking. Serve remaining sauce over chicken.

Nutrition Info: (Per Serving): 54 g water; 147 calories (12% from fat, 47% from protein, 40% from carb); 16 g protein; 2 g total fat; 1 g saturated fat; 1 g monounsaturated fat; 0 g polyunsaturated fat; 14 g carb; 0 g fiber; 12 g sugar; 17 mg calcium; 1 mg iron; 50 mg sodium; 157 mg potassium; 23 IU vitamin A; 1 mg vitamin C; 44 mg cholesterol

Roasted Lemon Chicken

Servings: 6

Ingredients:

- 6 (10-ounce) bone-in, skin-on chicken breasts
- 1 medium lemon
- 3 cloves garlic, thinly sliced
- 3 tablespoons Mustard
- 1 teaspoon dried thyme leaves
- 1/4 teaspoon white pepper

Directions:

1. Preheat oven to 400°F. Loosen skin from the chicken, leaving it attached. Thinly slice half of the lemon to get 6 slices.
2. Carefully stuff a lemon slice and a few garlic slices under the skin of each piece; smooth skin back over the meat.
3. Squeeze juice from remaining lemon half into a dish and mix in mustard; spread each chicken breast with this mixture, then sprinkle with thyme and pepper. Place chicken in roasting pan.

4. Roast chicken for 30–40 minutes or until a meat thermometer registers 160°F. Let stand for 5 minutes, then serve.

Nutrition Info: (Per Serving):Calories: 145; Total Fat: 2 g; Saturated Fat: 0 g; Cholesterol: 65 mg; Protein: 27 g; Sodium: 74 mg; Potassium: 325 mg; Fiber: 0 g; Carbohydrates: 2 g; Sugar: 0 g

Herbed Chicken Paprikash

Servings: 6

Ingredients:

- 4 (8-ounce) chicken leg quarters, skin removed
- Olive oil spray
- 1/4 teaspoon dried marjoram or oregano
- 1/4 teaspoon dried thyme
- 1/4 teaspoon dried basil
- 1/8 teaspoon dried rosemary
- 1/3 cup dry white wine
- 1/3 cup low-sodium chicken broth
- 2/3 cup fresh button mushrooms, sliced
- 1 clove garlic, minced
- 1/4 cup finely grated carrots
- 2 tablespoons unbleached all-purpose flour
- 2 tablespoons water
- 1 teaspoon paprika
- 2 tablespoons plain nonfat yogurt
- Optional: Additional paprika, for garnish

Directions:

1.   Bring a deep nonstick skillet to temperature over medium heat. Spray both sides of the chicken with the olive oil spray. Sprinkle the chicken with the marjoram or oregano, thyme, basil, and rosemary. Add the chicken to the skillet and cook for 2 minutes on each side or until browned.

2.   Add the wine and chicken broth to pan; bring to a boil. Reduce heat, cover, and simmer for 20 minutes. Add the mushrooms, garlic, and carrots, cover, and simmer for an additional 10 minutes or until chicken registers 160°F. Use tongs to transfer the chicken to a serving plate. Keep warm.

3.   In a small bowl, mix together the flour and water, whisking to remove any lumps. Add the mixture to the pan and increase heat to medium; bring to a boil, stirring constantly. Continue to cook over medium heat, stirring until the mixture thickens.

4.   Stir in the paprika. Remove from heat and stir in the yogurt. Pour the sauce over the

chicken. Sprinkle with additional paprika, if desired.

Nutrition Info: (Per Serving):Calories: 209; Total Fat: 5 g; Saturated Fat: 1 g; Cholesterol: 120 mg; Protein: 31 g; Sodium: 137 mg; Potassium: 412 mg; Fiber: 0 g; Carbohydrates: 3 g; Sugar: 0 g

Kay's Chicken Rice Bake

Servings: 6

Ingredients:

- 1 ½ cups (292 g) uncooked rice
- 1 ½ cups (355 ml) low sodium chicken broth
- 1 ½ cups (355 ml) water
- 12 ounces (340 g) frozen broccoli
- 6 chicken thighs
- For soup:
- ½ cup (125 g) frozen broccoli, chopped
- ½ cup (80 g) onion, chopped
- ¼ teaspoon garlic powder
- 1 tablespoon (0.4 g) dried parsley
- ½ cup (120 ml) low sodium chicken broth
- ⅔ cup (157 ml) skim milk
- 2 tablespoons (16 g) cornstarch

Directions:

1. To make soup: Cook broccoli, onion, and spices in chicken broth until soft. Process in a blender or food processor until well pureed. Shake together milk and cornstarch until dissolved. Cook and stir until thick. Stir in

46

veggie mixture. Mix together rice, soup, broth, and water in the bottom of a 9 × 13-inch (23 × 33-cm) roasting pan. Stir in remaining broccoli. Top with chicken pieces. Bake at 375°F (190°C, gas mark 5) until chicken is done and rice soft, about 1 hour.

Nutrition Info: (Per Serving): 302 g water; 152 calories (12% from fat, 35% from protein, 53% from carb); 14 g protein; 2 g total fat; 1 g saturated fat; 1 g monounsaturated fat; 1 g polyunsaturated fat; 20 g carb; 1 g fiber; 1 g sugar; 94 mg calcium; 2 mg iron; 141 mg sodium; 455 mg potassium; 1955 IU vitamin A; 60 mg vitamin C; 35 mg cholesterol

Sun-dried Tomato Coated Chicken

Servings: 2

Ingredients:

- 2 boneless chicken breasts
- ½ cup (60 g) low sodium bread crumbs
- ¼ cup (27.5 g) sun-dried tomatoes in oil
- 1 clove garlic, minced
- 1 egg
- 2 tablespoons (30 ml) olive oil

Directions:

1. Split chicken breasts in half to make two thin cutlets (or pound them flat, but that always seemed like wasted effort to me). Combine bread crumbs, tomatoes, and garlic in food processor. Process until well blended. Dip chicken in beaten eggs and then in crumb mixture to coat thoroughly. Heat oil in an ovenproof skillet. Brown chicken about 2 minutes on each side, until just golden brown. Transfer skillet to a preheated 400°F (200°C, gas mark 6) oven and cook until chicken is cooked through, about 10 minutes.

Nutrition Info: (Per Serving): 66 g water; 386 calories (51% from fat, 25% from protein, 24% from carb); 24 g protein; 22 g total fat; 4 g saturated fat; 13 g monounsaturated fat; 3 g polyunsaturated fat; 23 g carb; 2 g fiber; 2 g sugar; 82 mg calcium; 3 mg iron; 126 mg sodium; 446 mg potassium; 328 IU vitamin A; 14 mg vitamin C; 167 mg cholesterol

Country Captain–style Chicken

Servings: 6

Ingredients:

- 6 chicken thighs
- 2 cups (475 ml) no-salt-added tomatoes
- 1 onion, chopped
- ½ teaspoon garlic powder
- ½ cup (65 g) frozen peas
- 1 ½ tablespoons (7.3 g) curry powder

Directions:

1. Place chicken in a 9 × 13-inch (23 × 33-cm) baking dish. Mix other ingredients together and pour over chicken. Bake at 350°F (180°C, gas mark 4) until chicken is done, about 45 minutes.

Nutrition Info: (Per Serving): 135 g water; 89 calories (19% from fat, 43% from protein, 37% from carb); 10 g protein; 2 g total fat; 0 g saturated fat; 1 g monounsaturated fat; 1 g polyunsaturated fat; 9 g carb; 2 g fiber; 4 g sugar; 43 mg calcium; 2 mg iron; 54 mg sodium; 347 mg potassium; 427 IU vitamin A; 14 mg vitamin C; 34 mg cholesterol

Indoor-grilled Chicken Breast

Servings: 4

Ingredients:

- 1 teaspoon cider vinegar
- 1 teaspoon garlic powder
- 4 teaspoons salt-free honey mustard
- 1 teaspoon brown sugar
- 1 teaspoon Citrus Pepper
- 2 teaspoons olive oil
- 4 (4-ounce) boneless, skinless chicken breast cutlets

Directions:

1. In a medium-size bowl, combine the cider vinegar, garlic powder, honey mustard, brown sugar, and Citrus Pepper. Slowly whisk in the olive oil to thoroughly combine and make a paste.

2. Rinse the chicken cutlets and dry between paper towels. If necessary to ensure a uniform thickness of the cutlets, put them between sheets of plastic wrap or waxed paper and pound to flatten them.

3. Pour the marinade into a heavy-duty (freezer-style) sealable plastic bag. Add the chicken cutlets, moving them around in the mixture to coat all sides. Seal the bag, carefully squeezing out as much air as possible. Refrigerate and allow the chicken to marinate for at least 1 hour, or as long as overnight.

4. Preheat an indoor (George Foreman–style) grill. When the grill is heated, place the chicken on the grill. Close the grill lid and cook the cutlets for 3–4 minutes or until a food thermometer registers 160°F.

Nutrition Info: (Per Serving):Calories: 163; Total Fat: 4 g; Saturated Fat: 0 g; Cholesterol: 65 mg; Protein: 26 g; Sodium: 74 mg; Potassium: 311 mg; Fiber: 0 g; Carbohydrates: 3 g; Sugar: 2 g

Cobb Pita Sandwich

Servings: 4

Ingredients:

- 2 (6-ounce) boneless, skinless chicken breasts
- 1/2 teaspoon dried thyme leaves
- 1/8 teaspoon white pepper
- 1/4 cup lemon juice, divided
- 2 tablespoons olive oil
- 1/3 cup sour cream
- 2 tablespoons Mayonnaise
- 2 tablespoons Honey Mustard
- 2 Hard-Cooked Eggs , peeled and chopped
- 1 medium avocado, peeled and chopped
- 1/2 cup chopped fresh mushrooms
- 2 whole Pita Breads
- 1 cup torn butter lettuce

Directions:

1. Sprinkle chicken breasts with thyme and pepper and 1 tablespoon lemon juice; set aside for 10 minutes.
2. Heat olive oil in medium saucepan over medium heat. Sauté chicken, turning once,

until light brown and thoroughly cooked to 160°F, about 8–9 minutes. Remove from pan, cover with foil, and let stand for 10 minutes.

3.   In large bowl, combine remaining lemon juice, sour cream, mayonnaise, and honey mustard and mix well.

4.   Cut chicken into cubes and add to dressing in bowl. Add eggs, avocado, and mushrooms.

5.   Cut the pita breads in half and open pockets. Line each pocket with lettuce and fill with chicken mixture; serve immediately.

Nutrition Info: (Per Serving):Calories: 450; Total Fat: 6 g; Saturated Fat: 30 g; Cholesterol: 157 mg; Protein: 21 g; Sodium: 97 mg; Potassium: 569 mg; Fiber: 4 g; Carbohydrates: 25 g; Sugar: 5 g

Turkey Burgers

Servings: 4

Ingredients:

- 1 tablespoon olive oil
- 1 small onion, diced
- 3 cloves garlic, minced
- 2 tablespoons Chicken Stock or water
- 2 tablespoons Honey Mustard
- 1 tablespoon lemon juice
- 11/4 pounds ground turkey
- 1 large red bell pepper
- 1/4 cup Mayonnaise
- 4 Hamburger Buns , split and toasted
- 2 medium avocados, sliced

Directions:

1. In small saucepan, heat olive oil over medium heat. Add onion; cook for 5 minutes, stirring frequently. Add garlic; cook for another 1–2 minutes until vegetables are tender. Remove from heat and place in large bowl.

2. Add chicken stock, honey mustard, and lemon juice to vegetables and stir. Add turkey

and mix with hands. Form into 4 burgers; cover and refrigerate.

3. Hold the red bell pepper over a gas flame, or broil it, until the skin is blackened. Put the pepper into a paper bag and close; let stand 5 minutes. Peel skin off pepper and discard. Cut pepper into strips and remove seeds.

4. Prepare and preheat grill. Cook burgers for 7–9 minutes, turning once, until they register 165°F on a meat thermometer. Remove from grill.

5. To assemble burgers, spread mayonnaise on the hamburger buns. Place turkey burgers on bun bottoms, then add bell pepper strips, and avocado. Add bun tops and serve immediately.

Nutrition Info: (Per Serving):Calories: 801; Total Fat: 48 g; Saturated Fat: 6 g; Cholesterol: 122 mg; Protein: 36 g; Sodium: 129 mg; Potassium: 734 mg; Fiber: 10 g; Carbohydrates: 64 g; Sugar: 12 g

Mustard-braised Chicken

Servings: 4

Ingredients:

- 8 bone-in, skin-on chicken thighs
- 1/8 teaspoon pepper
- 1 teaspoon dry mustard powder
- 1 teaspoon dried basil leaves
- 1 tablespoon unsalted butter
- 1 tablespoon olive oil
- 1 medium onion, chopped
- 3 cloves garlic, sliced
- 2 russet potatoes, cut into 11/2" pieces
- 11/2 cups Chicken Stock
- 6 tablespoons Grainy Mustard , divided
- 2 tablespoons chopped chives

Directions:

1. Sprinkle chicken with pepper, mustard powder, and basil; rub into skin and set aside for 10 minutes.

2. Combine butter and olive oil in a large skillet with a lid over medium heat. Add chicken, skin-side down; cook until browned, about 5–6 minutes. Remove chicken to plate.

3.   Add onion and garlic to skillet; cook, stirring to remove pan drippings, until onion is crisp-tender, about 5–6 minutes.
4.   Return chicken to skillet and place potatoes around chicken.
5.   In small bowl, combine stock and 4 tablespoons mustard; mix well. Pour into skillet.
6.   Bring to a simmer over medium heat, then reduce heat to low. Cover and simmer until chicken registers 160°F on a thermometer and potatoes are tender. Stir in remaining mustard, then sprinkle with chives and serve.

Nutrition Info: (Per Serving):Calories: 564; Total Fat: 28 g; Saturated Fat: 7 g; Cholesterol: 122 mg; Protein: 37 g; Sodium: 128 mg; Potassium: 1,190 mg; Fiber: 4 g; Carbohydrates: 37 g; Sugar: 3 g

Slow Cooker Chicken Paprikash

Servings: 4

Ingredients:

- 8 (4-ounce) boneless, skinless chicken thighs, cut into 1" strips
- 1 (8-ounce) package mushrooms, sliced
- 1 medium onion, chopped
- 4 cloves garlic, sliced
- 1 tablespoon sweet paprika
- 1 tablespoon smoked paprika
- 3 tablespoons tomato paste
- 1 (14-ounce) can no-salt-added fire-roasted diced tomatoes, undrained
- 1/2 cup Chicken Stock
- 2 tablespoons lemon juice
- 2 tablespoons flour
- 2/3 cup sour cream

Directions:

1. In 4- to 5-quart slow cooker, combine chicken, mushrooms, onion, and garlic and mix. Sprinkle with both kinds of paprika and toss to coat.

2.   In medium bowl, combine tomato paste, diced tomatoes, chicken stock, and lemon juice and mix well. Pour into slow cooker.

3.   Cover and cook on low for 6–8 hours or until chicken is cooked to 165°F and is tender.

4.   In small bowl, combine flour and sour cream and mix with wire whisk. Ladle 1/3 cup of the liquid from the slow cooker into the sour-cream mixture and mix well. Stir into slow cooker; cover and cook on high for about 10 minutes or until sauce is thickened. Serve over hot cooked rice or noodles.

Nutrition Info: (Per Serving):Calories: 246; Total Fat: 11 g; Saturated Fat: 5 g; Cholesterol: 87 mg; Protein: 21 g; Sodium: 136 mg; Potassium: 872 mg; Fiber: 3 g; Carbohydrates: 16 g; Sugar: 6 g

Easy Italian-seasoned Turkey Sausage

Servings: 8

Ingredients:

- 1 pound lean ground turkey
- 11/2 teaspoons salt-free seasoning blend

Directions:

1. In a mixing bowl, combine the ground turkey with your choice of seasoning blend until well mixed. Form into 8 equal-sized patties.

2. Pan-fry in a nonstick grill pan or prepare in a covered indoor grill (such as a George Foreman–style indoor grill). The sausage is done when the temperature registers 165°F.

Nutrition Info: (Per Serving):Calories: 75; Total Fat: 3 g; Saturated Fat: 0 g; Cholesterol: 0 mg; Protein: 11 g; Sodium: 40 mg; Potassium: 0 mg; Fiber: 0 g; Carbohydrates: 0 g; Sugar: 0 g

Chicken And Mushroom Risotto

Servings: 6

Ingredients:

- 1 ounce dried mushrooms
- 1/2 cup warm water
- 3 (6-ounce) boneless, skinless chicken breasts
- 2 tablespoons unsalted butter
- 1 tablespoon olive oil
- 1 medium onion, chopped
- 4 cloves garlic, minced
- 1 (8-ounce) package button mushrooms, sliced
- 11/2 cups uncooked Arborio or long-grain rice
- 1/2 cup dry white wine
- 3–4 cups Chicken Stock
- 1/3 cup crumbled soft goat cheese
- 2 tablespoons minced fresh chives

Directions:

1. Place dried mushrooms in a small bowl and cover with water; let stand until softened. Drain mushrooms, reserving liquid. Cut stems

62

off mushrooms and discard; chop mushrooms. Strain liquid and set aside.

2. Cut chicken into 1" cubes and set aside.

3. Heat unsalted butter and olive oil in a large saucepan over medium heat. Add onion and garlic; cook for 3 minutes.

4. Add button mushrooms; cook for 5–7 minutes longer or until mushrooms give up their liquid and the liquid evaporates. Stir in chicken; cook for 3 minutes. Add rehydrated dried mushrooms.

5. Add the rice; cook and stir for 2 minutes. Then add the reserved mushroom soaking liquid and wine; cook over medium heat, stirring frequently, until liquid is absorbed.

6. Add the chicken stock, one ladle at a time, stirring after each addition, until the rice is tender. This should take about 20–25 minutes. Add the goat cheese and chives.

7. Cover and remove from heat; let stand for 3–4 minutes. Stir and serve immediately.

Nutrition Info: (Per Serving):Calories: 413; Total Fat: 14 g; Saturated Fat: 6 g; Cholesterol: 94 mg; Protein:

37 g; Sodium: 135 mg; Potassium: 592 mg; Fiber: 1 g; Carbohydrates: 28 g; Sugar: 1 g

Beer Can Chicken

Servings: 8

Ingredients:

- 1 chicken, 4 to 6 pounds (1 ¾ to 2 ¾ kg)
- 3 tablespoons Memphis Rub
- 1 can(12 ounces) beer
- 3 cloves garlic

Directions:

1. Remove and discard the fat from inside the body cavities of the chicken. Remove the package of giblets and set aside for another use. Rinse the chicken, inside and out, under cold running water; then drain and blot dry, inside and out, with paper towels. Sprinkle 1 tablespoon of the rub inside the body and neck cavities; then rub the rest all over the skin of the bird. If you wish, rub another half-tablespoon of the mixture between the flesh and the skin. Cover and refrigerate the chicken while you preheat the grill.

2. Pop the tab on the beer can. Using a "church key" type of can opener, punch 6 or 7 holes in the top of the can. Pour out the top inch (5

cm) of beer; drop the peeled garlic cloves into the holes in the can. Holding the chicken upright (wings at top, legs at bottom) with the opening of the body cavity down, insert the beer can into the lower cavity. Oil the grill grate. Stand the chicken up in the center of the hot grate, over the drip pan. Spread out the legs to form a sort of tripod, to support the bird. Cover the grill and cook the chicken until fall-off-the-bone tender, about an hour, depending on size. Use a thermometer to check for doneness. The internal temperature should be 180°F (82°C). Using tongs, lift the bird to a cutting board or platter, holding a metal spatula underneath the beer can for support.

Nutrition Info: (Per Serving): 25 g water; 81 calories (66% from fat, 32% from protein, 2% from carb); 6 g protein; 6 g total fat; 2 g saturated fat; 2 g monounsaturated fat; 1 g polyunsaturated fat; 0 g carb; 0 g fiber; 0 g sugar; 6 mg calcium; 0 mg iron; 25 mg sodium; 76 mg potassium; 48 IU vitamin A; 0 mg vitamin C; 27 mg cholesterol

Easy Chicken Barbecue

Servings: 4

Ingredients:

- 1 tablespoon water or chicken broth or lemon juice
- 1 small sweet onion, chopped
- 1 clove garlic, chopped
- 1 pound Seasoned Chicken
- 1/4 cup no-salt-added honey barbecue sauce and marinade

Directions:

1. In a medium-size microwave-safe bowl, combine the water, onion, and garlic; microwave on high for 3 minutes or until the onion is transparent.
2. Add the chicken and barbecue sauce to the bowl; mix well. Cover and microwave at 70 percent power for 2 minutes or until the chicken is heated through; stir and serve.

Nutrition Info: (Per Serving):Calories: 138; Total Fat: 4 g; Saturated Fat: 1 g; Cholesterol: 90 mg; Protein: 22 g; Sodium: 107 mg; Potassium: 267 mg; Fiber: 0 g; Carbohydrates: 0 g; Sugar: 0 g

Chicken With Mostarda

Servings: 4

Ingredients:

- 4 (6-ounce) boneless, skinless chicken breasts
- 1/8 teaspoon white pepper
- 1/2 teaspoon grated lemon zest
- 11/4 cups Mostarda

Directions:

1. Prepare and preheat grill. While the grill is heating, sprinkle chicken with pepper and lemon zest.
2. When ready to grill, pound the chicken breasts until they are an even thickness, about 1/3" thick.
3. Drain off some of the liquid from the Mostarda and place in a small cup.
4. Place chicken on grill over medium-high heat and brush with liquid from Mostarda. Grill for 2–3 minutes on each side, turning once and brushing again with the liquid, until done to 160°F.

5. Remove chicken from grill; discard remaining Mostarda liquid. Serve chicken with remaining Mostarda.

Nutrition Info: (Per Serving):Calories: 377; Total Fat: 3 g; Saturated Fat: 0 g; Cholesterol: 65 mg; Protein: 29 g; Sodium: 85 mg; Potassium: 746 mg; Fiber: 5 g; Carbohydrates: 58 g; Sugar: 48 g

Chicken Salad

Servings: 4

Ingredients:

- 1 cup (110 g) chicken, cooked
- ¼ cup (25 g) celery, chopped
- 2 tablespoons (28 g) low sodium mayonnaise
- 2 tablespoons (30 g) sour cream
- ½ teaspoon onion powder

Directions:

1. Place chicken and celery in food processor and process until finely ground. Add remaining ingredients and process until well mixed.

Nutrition Info: (Per Serving): 36 g water; 133 calories (65% from fat, 32% from protein, 3% from carb); 11 g protein; 10 g total fat; 2 g saturated fat; 3 g monounsaturated fat; 3 g polyunsaturated fat; 1 g carb; 0 g fiber; 0 g sugar; 19 mg calcium; 0 mg iron; 42 mg sodium; 120 mg potassium; 118 IU vitamin A; 0 mg vitamin C; 38 mg cholesterol

Pineapple Curry Chicken

Servings: 4

Ingredients:

- 1 medium onion, chopped
- 1 cup baby carrots
- 3 cloves garlic, minced
- 4 (6-ounce) boneless, skinless chicken breasts, cut into strips
- 2 (8-ounce) cans pineapple tidbits, drained, reserving juice
- 1 tablespoon curry powder
- 1 (13-ounce) can coconut milk
- 1/2 cup Chicken Stock
- 2 tablespoons cornstarch
- 2 tablespoons water

Directions:

1. In 4- to 5-quart slow cooker, place onion, carrots, and garlic. Top with chicken breasts, then add pineapple.
2. In small bowl, combine curry powder with reserved pineapple liquid; pour into slow cooker. Add coconut milk and stock.

3. Cover and cook on low for 7–8 hours or until chicken is tender and thoroughly cooked to 160°F.

4. In small bowl, combine cornstarch and water and mix until smooth. Stir into slow cooker; cover and cook on high for 10–15 minutes or until sauce is thickened. Serve over hot cooked rice.

Nutrition Info: (Per Serving):Calories: 416; Total Fat: 21 g; Saturated Fat: 17 g; Cholesterol: 65 mg; Protein: 29 g; Sodium: 119 mg; Potassium: 798 mg; Fiber: 3 g; Carbohydrates: 29 g; Sugar: 17 g

Polynesian Chicken

Servings: 4

Ingredients:

- 8 ounces (225 g) pineapple chunks
- ¼ cup (85 g) honey
- ¼ cup (60 ml) red wine vinegar
- 4 chicken thighs
- ½ cup (60 g) red bell pepper, chopped
- ½ cup (80 g) onion, coarsely chopped

Directions:

1. Drain pineapple, reserving juice. Combine juice, honey, and vinegar. Place chicken in an 8 × 13-inch (20 × 33-cm) baking pan. Sprinkle pineapple and vegetables over top. Pour juice mixture over. Bake at 350°F (180°C, gas mark 4) until chicken is done, about 45 minutes.

Nutrition Info: (Per Serving): 126 g water; 144 calories (10% from fat, 23% from protein, 67% from carb); 9 g protein; 2 g total fat; 0 g saturated fat; 1 g monounsaturated fat; 0 g polyunsaturated fat; 26 g carb; 1 g fiber; 24 g sugar; 20 mg calcium; 1 mg iron;

38 mg sodium; 241 mg potassium; 337 IU vitamin A; 23 mg vitamin C; 34 mg cholesterol

Easy Ginger Cashew Chicken And Broccoli

Servings: 4

Ingredients:

- 1 tablespoon water or chicken broth or lemon juice
- 1 small sweet onion, chopped
- 1 clove garlic, chopped
- 4 cups broccoli florets
- 1 pound cooked dark-meat chicken, chopped
- 6 tablespoons salt-free ginger stir-fry sauce
- 1/4 cup unsalted dry-roasted cashew pieces
- Optional: Candied ginger, minced

Directions:

1. In a large microwave-safe bowl, combine the water, onion, garlic, and broccoli. Cover and microwave on high for 4 minutes or until the broccoli is crisp-tender.

2. Add the chicken and stir-fry sauce; stir well. Microwave at 70 percent power for 2 minutes or until the mixture is heated through.

3. Serve over cooked rice; top each serving with 1 tablespoon of the cashews, and minced candied ginger, if desired.

Nutrition Info: (Per Serving):Calories: 235; Total Fat: 9 g; Saturated Fat: 2 g; Cholesterol: 90 mg; Protein: 26 g; Sodium: 118 mg; Potassium: 542 mg; Fiber: 0 g; Carbohydrates: 13 g; Sugar: 2 g

Cajun-style Chicken

Servings: 4

Ingredients:

- 4 (4-ounce) boneless, skinless chicken breasts
- 2 teaspoons olive oil
- 1/2 teaspoon paprika
- 1/2 teaspoon cayenne pepper
- 1/4 teaspoon onion powder
- 1/4 teaspoon garlic powder
- 1/4 teaspoon freshly ground black pepper
- 1/4 teaspoon freshly ground white pepper
- 1/8 teaspoon dried oregano
- 1/8 teaspoon dried thyme
- 1/8 teaspoon dried basil
- 1/8 teaspoon dried rosemary
- Optional: 1/4 teaspoon brown sugar

Directions:

1. Put the chicken breasts and olive oil in a heavy-duty, sealable plastic bag. Turn the bag to completely coat the chicken in the oil.

2. In a medium bowl, mix together the remaining ingredients. Dip the top half of each chicken breast in the dried seasoning mixture.

3. Heat a nonstick skillet or grill pan on medium-high. Place the chicken breasts in the skillet, spice-coated-side down. Cook for 2–3 minutes or until the top half of the chicken begins to lose its pinkish color and the spiced side of the chicken is browned well. Use tongs to turn the chicken. Cook for 2–3 minutes longer or until the chicken is done to 160°F.

Nutrition Info: (Per Serving):Calories: 147; Total Fat: 3 g; Saturated Fat: 0 g; Cholesterol: 65 mg; Protein: 26 g; Sodium: 73 mg; Potassium: 305 mg; Fiber: 0 g; Carbohydrates: 0 g; Sugar: 0 g

Yogurt "fried" Chicken

Servings: 4

Ingredients:

- Olive oil spray
- 4 (1-ounce) slices French Bread
- 1 pound boneless, skinless chicken breasts (trimmed of fat)
- 1 teaspoon garlic powder
- 1 teaspoon paprika
- 1/4 teaspoon mustard powder
- 1/4 teaspoon dried thyme
- 2 teaspoons Citrus Pepper
- 1 cup nonfat plain yogurt

Directions:

1. Preheat oven to 350°F. Treat a baking pan with the olive oil spray.
2. Place the bread in the bowl of a food processor or in a blender; process to make bread crumbs.
3. Cut the chicken breasts into 8 equal-sized strips.

4. In a medium-size bowl, combine the garlic powder, paprika, mustard powder, thyme, and Citrus Pepper with the yogurt and mix well.

5. Add the chicken to the yogurt mixture, stirring to make sure all sides of the strips are covered. Lift the chicken strips out of the yogurt mixture and dredge all sides in the bread crumbs. Lightly mist the breaded chicken pieces with the spray oil and arrange in the pan.

6. Bake for 10 minutes. Use a spatula or tongs to turn the chicken pieces. Optional: For the last 5 minutes of cooking, place the pan under the broiler to give the chicken a deep golden color. Watch closely to ensure the chicken "crust" doesn't burn.

Nutrition Info: (Per Serving):Calories: 244; Total Fat: 2 g; Saturated Fat: 0 g; Cholesterol: 66 mg; Protein: 31 g; Sodium: 136 mg; Potassium: 501 mg; Fiber: 0 g; Carbohydrates: 21 g; Sugar: 5 g

Rotisserie Chicken

Servings: 8

Ingredients:

- 1 teaspoon paprika
- 1 teaspoon onion powder
- ½ teaspoon black pepper
- ½ teaspoon dried thyme
- ¼ teaspoon garlic powder
- ¼ cup (85 g) honey
- 1 large roasting chicken (6 to 7 pounds, or 2 ½ to 3 ¼ kg)

Directions:

1. Mix spices into honey. Brush onto chicken. Roast at 325°F (170°C, gas mark 3) until done, basting occasionally with pan juices.

Nutrition Info: (Per Serving): 16 g water; 71 calories (18% from fat, 30% from protein, 51% from carb); 5 g protein; 1 g total fat; 0 g saturated fat; 1 g monounsaturated fat; 0 g polyunsaturated fat; 9 g carb; 0 g fiber; 9 g sugar; 7 mg calcium; 0 mg iron; 17 mg sodium; 67 mg potassium; 163 IU vitamin A; 0 mg vitamin C; 16 mg cholesterol

Chicken Strips

Servings: 4

Ingredients:

- 1 pound (455 g) boneless chicken breast
- ¼ cup (28 g) all-purpose flour
- ¼ cup (35 g) cornmeal
- ½ teaspoon black pepper
- 1 teaspoon Dick's Salt-Free Seasoning
- ¼ teaspoon poultry seasoning
- 1 egg, beaten
- Nonstick vegetable oil spray

Directions:

1. Cut chicken into strips. Combine flour, cornmeal, and spices. Roll chicken first in egg, then in flour mixture. Repeat. Place chicken on baking sheet sprayed with nonstick vegetable oil spray. Spray chicken with spray until all is moistened. Bake at 350°F (180°C, gas mark 4) until done, 20 to 30 minutes, turning once.

Nutrition Info: (Per Serving): 21 g water; 104 calories (19% from fat, 29% from protein, 51% from carb); 7 g protein; 2 g total fat; 1 g saturated fat; 1 g monounsaturated fat; 0 g polyunsaturated fat; 13 g carb; 1 g fiber; 0 g sugar; 13 mg calcium; 1 mg iron; 30 mg sodium; 79 mg potassium; 94 IU vitamin A; 0 mg vitamin C; 72 mg cholesterol

Curried Turkey Burgers

Servings: 4

Ingredients:

- 1 tablespoon olive oil
- 2 scallions, minced
- 2 cloves garlic, minced
- 1 tablespoon minced fresh ginger root
- 21/2 teaspoons curry powder, divided
- 11/4 pounds ground turkey
- 1/3 cup sour cream
- 1/3 cup Mango Chutney
- 1 tablespoon lemon juice
- 1/8 teaspoon white pepper
- 4 Hamburger Buns , split and toasted
- 4 leaves butter lettuce
- 1/2 cup sliced cucumbers

Directions:

1. In small saucepan, heat olive oil over medium heat. Add scallions, garlic, and ginger root; cook and stir for 3–4 minutes until fragrant. Add 2 teaspoons curry powder and cook for 30 seconds; remove to large bowl and let cool.

2. Add turkey to vegetables and mix with your hands. Form into 4 patties and refrigerate.

3. In small bowl, combine sour cream, chutney, lemon juice, remaining 1/2 teaspoon curry powder, and white pepper and refrigerate.

4. When ready to eat, prepare and preheat grill. Grill burgers, turning once, until they register 165°F on a meat thermometer, about 8–10 minutes.

5. Spread the chutney mixture on the bottom half of the hamburger buns. Add lettuce, cucumbers, turkey burgers, and bun tops, then serve immediately.

Nutrition Info: (Per Serving):Calories: 562; Total Fat: 23 g; Saturated Fat: 4 g; Cholesterol: 102 mg; Protein: 30 g; Sodium: 137 mg; Potassium: 244 mg; Fiber: 3 g; Carbohydrates: 58 g; Sugar: 14 g

Crunchy Flaxseed Chicken

Servings: 4

Ingredients:

- 4 (6-ounce) boneless, skinless chicken breasts
- 1/2 cup ground flaxseeds
- 3 tablespoons sesame seeds
- 3 tablespoons flour
- 1/2 teaspoon dried marjoram leaves
- 1/8 teaspoon white pepper
- 3 tablespoons Mayonnaise
- 1 tablespoon Mustard
- 1 egg white
- 2 tablespoons unsalted butter
- 1 tablespoon olive oil

Directions:

1. Place chicken breasts on a platter. On another platter, combine flaxseeds, sesame seeds, flour, marjoram, and white pepper. On a shallow plate, combine mayonnaise, mustard, and egg white and beat well.
2. Dip the chicken into the mayonnaise mixture, shake off excess, then dip into the

flaxseed mixture to coat well. Refrigerate chicken for 15 minutes.

3.   When ready to eat, melt butter and olive oil in a large skillet over medium heat. Add chicken and cook for 10–14 minutes, turning once, until a meat thermometer registers 160°F. Serve immediately.

Nutrition Info: (Per Serving):Calories: 460; Total Fat: 31 g; Saturated Fat: 7 g; Cholesterol: 94 mg; Protein: 32 g; Sodium: 97 mg; Potassium: 506 mg; Fiber: 6 g; Carbohydrates: 12 g; Sugar: 0 g

Sticky Chicken

Servings: 8

Ingredients:

- 1 teaspoon cayenne pepper
- 1 teaspoon onion powder
- 1 teaspoon dried thyme
- 1 teaspoon white pepper
- ½ teaspoon black pepper
- ½ teaspoon garlic powder
- ½ teaspoon chili powder
- 1 chicken, the larger the better

Directions:

1. Combine the spices in a small bowl. Remove the giblets and neck from the chicken. Wash and dry the chicken inside and out. Rub the spices into the chicken inside and out, making sure to rub deep into the skin. Place the chicken in a sealed zip-top plastic bag and allow to sit in the refrigerator overnight. When ready to roast, remove the chicken from the bag and place in a roasting pan. Roast at 250°F (120°C, gas mark ½) for 5 hours. (Yes ... that low, that long.) Ignore the pop-up

timer if it has one. After the first hour, baste the chicken with the pan juices every half hour. At the end of roasting, remove the chicken from the oven and let stand 10 minutes before carving.

Nutrition Info: (Per Serving): 19 g water; 34 calories (23% from fat, 66% from protein, 11% from carb); 5 g protein; 1 g total fat; 0 g saturated fat; 0 g monounsaturated fat; 0 g polyunsaturated fat; 1 g carb; 0 g fiber; 0 g sugar; 9 mg calcium; 1 mg iron; 20 mg sodium; 71 mg potassium; 156 IU vitamin A; 1 mg vitamin C; 17 mg cholesterol

Slow-cooker Curried Chicken

Servings: 5

Ingredients:

- 5 medium potatoes, diced
- 1 green bell pepper, coarsely chopped
- 1 medium onion, coarsely chopped
- 1 pound (455 g) boneless chicken breast, cubed
- 2 cups (475 ml) no-salt-added tomatoes
- 1 tablespoon (6 g) coriander
- 1 ½ tablespoons (10.5 g) paprika
- 1 tablespoon (5.5 g) ground ginger
- ¼ teaspoon cayenne pepper
- ½ teaspoon turmeric
- ¼ teaspoon ground cinnamon
- ⅛ teaspoon cloves
- 1 cup (235 ml) low sodium chicken broth
- 2 tablespoons (28 ml) cold water
- 4 tablespoons (32 g) cornstarch

Directions:

1. Place vegetables in slow cooker. Place chicken on top. Mix together tomatoes, spices, and chicken broth. Pour over chicken. Cook on

low for 8 to 10 hours or on high for 5 to 6 hours. Remove meat and vegetables. Turn heat to high. Stir cornstarch into water. Add to slow cooker. Cook until sauce is slightly thickened, 15 to 20 minutes.

Nutrition Info: (Per Serving): 433 g water; 346 calories (3% from fat, 12% from protein, 85% from carb); 11 g protein; 1 g total fat; 0 g saturated fat; 0 g monounsaturated fat; 0 g polyunsaturated fat; 76 g carb; 8 g fiber; 7 g sugar; 77 mg calcium; 3 mg iron; 55 mg sodium; 1432 mg potassium; 1363 IU vitamin A; 65 mg vitamin C; 9 mg cholesterol

Red And Green Bell Pepper Chicken

Servings: 4

Ingredients:

- 4 teaspoons olive oil
- 1 medium green bell pepper, seeded and chopped
- 1 medium red bell pepper, seeded and chopped
- 2 cloves garlic, minced
- 4 (4-ounce) boneless, skinless chicken thighs
- 1/4 teaspoon freshly ground black pepper
- 2 tablespoons dry red or white wine
- 1 (14.5-ounce) can no-salt-added diced tomatoes
- 1 teaspoon dried basil
- 1/2 teaspoon dried parsley
- 1/8 teaspoon dried marjoram or oregano
- 1 teaspoon lemon juice
- 1/4 teaspoon granulated sugar

Directions:

1. Heat a deep nonstick skillet over medium heat. Add the olive oil and chopped bell

peppers; sauté until tender. Add the garlic and sauté for 1 minute, being careful not to burn the garlic. Push the mixture to the edges of the pan.

2.   Add the chicken thighs. Sprinkle the pepper over the chicken. Pan-fry for 2 minutes on each side. Use tongs to transfer the chicken to a bowl or platter; set aside.

3.   Add the wine to the pan. Bring to a boil and cook for 2 minutes, stirring the wine into the vegetables and using a spoon or spatula to scrape (deglaze) the bottom of the pan.

4.   Add the tomatoes, basil, parsley, marjoram or oregano, lemon juice, and sugar to the pan; stir to combine.

5.   Add the chicken back to the pan, spooning some of the tomatoes over the top of the chicken. Reduce heat. Simmer, covered, for 20–25 minutes or until chicken registers 165°F. Serve immediately.

Nutrition Info: (Per Serving):Calories: 217; Total Fat: 9 g; Saturated Fat: 1 g; Cholesterol: 94 mg; Protein: 23 g; Sodium: 110 mg; Potassium: 584 mg; Fiber: 2 g; Carbohydrates: 8 g; Sugar: 4 g

Apple-smoked Turkey Breast

Servings: 12

Ingredients:

- ½ cup (120 ml) apple juice
- 3 pounds (1 ¼ kg) turkey breast

Directions:

1. Inject the apple juice into the breast. Smoke until done, 6 to 8 hours. Fruit wood chips preferred.

Nutrition Info: (Per Serving): 93 g water; 131 calories (5% from fat, 91% from protein, 4% from carb); 28 g protein; 1 g total fat; 0 g saturated fat; 0 g monounsaturated fat; 0 g polyunsaturated fat; 1 g carb; 0 g fiber; 1 g sugar; 12 mg calcium; 1 mg iron; 56 mg sodium; 345 mg potassium; 0 IU vitamin A; 0 mg vitamin C; 70 mg cholesterol

Greek Chicken

Servings: 4

Ingredients:

- 4 (6-ounce) boneless, skinless chicken breasts
- 3 tablespoons olive oil
- 3 tablespoons lemon juice
- 2 cloves garlic, minced
- 1 tablespoon chopped fresh oregano
- 2 tablespoons chopped fresh mint
- 1 cup grape tomatoes, cut in half
- 1/2 cup Chicken Stock
- 1 tablespoon unsalted butter

Directions:

1. Place chicken in a resealable plastic bag. Add olive oil, lemon juice, garlic, oregano, and mint to the bag and seal. Massage chicken in the bag. Then place the bag in a baking dish and refrigerate at least 8 hours or overnight.

2. When you're ready to eat, heat a large saucepan over medium heat. Remove chicken from marinade; reserve marinade.

3. Add chicken to pan and cook, turning once, until cooked to 160°F, about 9–10 minutes. Remove chicken from pan and cover to keep warm.
4. Add tomatoes, reserved marinade, and chicken stock to pan and bring to a simmer. Simmer for 3–4 minutes until slightly reduced.
5. Remove pan from heat and swirl in butter. Place chicken on serving platter, pour sauce over, and serve immediately.

Nutrition Info: (Per Serving):Calories: 258; Total Fat: 14 g; Saturated Fat: 3 g; Cholesterol: 73 mg; Protein: 27 g; Sodium: 85 mg; Potassium: 449 mg; Fiber: 0 g; Carbohydrates: 3 g; Sugar: 1 g

Chicken Carbonara

Servings: 8

Ingredients:

- 4 (6-ounce) boneless, skinless chicken breasts, cubed
- 1/8 teaspoon white pepper
- 2 tablespoons unsalted butter
- 1 (16-ounce) package spaghetti
- 1 tablespoon olive oil
- 1 medium onion, chopped
- 1 medium red bell pepper, chopped
- 3 cloves garlic, minced
- 4 large eggs, beaten
- 2/3 cup whole milk
- 1/4 cup grated Parmesan cheese

Directions:

1. Bring a large pot of water to a boil over high heat.
2. Sprinkle chicken with pepper. In large skillet, melt butter over medium heat. Add chicken; cook, stirring frequently, until chicken registers 160°F on a meat thermometer. Remove chicken from skillet and set aside.

3. Add pasta to water; cook according to package directions until al dente, or just barely tender to the bite.
4. Meanwhile, add olive oil to skillet; cook onion, bell pepper, and garlic until tender, about 4–5 minutes. Return chicken to skillet and remove from heat.
5. In medium bowl, beat eggs with milk and cheese.
6. Reserve 1/2 cup pasta-cooking water. Drain pasta and immediately add to skillet with chicken and vegetables.
7. Pour egg mixture over hot pasta and chicken mixture and toss with tongs until coated, adding some of the reserved pasta-cooking water if needed to form a smooth sauce. Serve immediately.

Nutrition Info: (Per Serving):Calories: 472; Total Fat: 12 g; Saturated Fat: 4 g; Cholesterol: 191 mg; Protein: 40 g; Sodium: 125 mg; Potassium: 346 mg; Fiber: 3 g; Carbohydrates: 45 g; Sugar: 2 g

Buffalo Chicken Thighs

Servings: 6

Ingredients:

- 5 chicken thighs, skinned
- 2 tablespoons (28 g) unsalted butter
- 3 tablespoons hot pepper sauce
- 2 tablespoons (30 ml) white vinegar

Directions:

1. Grill thighs over medium coals, turning frequently until done, about 30 minutes. Melt butter in a small saucepan; add the hot pepper sauce and white vinegar. Place the chicken In a large resealable plastic bag. Pour the mixture over the chicken, seal, and shake to coat. Remove, allowing extra sauce to drain.

Nutrition Info: (Per Serving): 38 g water; 76 calories (62% from fat, 36 % from protein, 2% from carb); 7 g protein; 5 g total fat; 3 g saturated fat; 1 g monounsaturated fat; 1 g polyunsaturated fat; 0 g carb; 0 g fiber; 0 g sugar; 6 mg calcium; 0 mg iron; 75 mg sodium; 94 mg potassium; 256 IU vitamin A; 0 mg vitamin C; 39 mg cholesterol

Chicken Chutney Stir-fry

Servings: 4

Ingredients:

- 3 (6-ounce) boneless, skinless chicken breasts, cubed
- 2 teaspoons curry powder
- 1/8 teaspoon white pepper
- 3/4 cup coconut milk
- 1/4 cup mango chutney
- 1 tablespoon cornstarch
- 2 tablespoons safflower oil
- 1 medium onion, chopped
- 1 large carrot, cut into 1/4" rounds
- 1 medium yellow bell pepper, chopped
- 2 cloves garlic, minced
- 1/2 cup chopped unsalted peanuts

Directions:

1. In bowl, combine chicken, curry powder, and white pepper; mix until coated. Set aside for 10 minutes.
2. In another bowl, combine coconut milk, chutney, and cornstarch and mix well.

3.   In wok or skillet, heat safflower oil over medium-high heat. Add chicken; stir-fry until chicken is almost done. Remove chicken from wok to a plate.

4.   Add onion to wok; stir-fry until crisp-tender, about 4 minutes. Add carrot; stir-fry for another 3 minutes. Add bell pepper and garlic; stir-fry for 2 minutes longer.

5.   Return chicken to wok. Add coconut-milk mixture; stir-fry until sauce is thickened and chicken is cooked to 160°F, about 3 minutes. Sprinkle with peanuts and serve with hot rice.

Nutrition Info: (Per Serving):Calories: 394; Total Fat: 26 g; Saturated Fat: 10 g; Cholesterol: 49 mg; Protein: 25 g; Sodium: 76 mg; Potassium: 640 mg; Fiber: 3 g; Carbohydrates: 17 g; Sugar: 5 g

Chicken Nuggets

Servings: 4

Ingredients:

- 1 pound (455 g) boneless chicken breast
- ½ cup (19 g) cornflakes, crushed
- 2 tablespoons nonfat dry milk
- 1 tablespoon (0.4 g) dried parsley
- 1 tablespoon (7 g) paprika
- 1 teaspoon onion powder
- ¼ teaspoon garlic powder
- ½ teaspoon poultry seasoning
- 1 egg, beaten

Directions:

1. Cut chicken into nugget-size pieces. Mix together cornflakes, dry milk, and spices in a resealable plastic bag. Dip chicken pieces in egg, then place in bag. Shake to coat evenly. Place on baking sheet sprayed with nonstick vegetable oil spray. Bake at 350°F (180°C, gas mark 4) until chicken is done and coating is crispy, about 20 minutes.

Nutrition Info: (Per Serving): 97 g water; 174 calories (17% from fat, 70% from protein, 13% from carb); 29

g protein; 3 g total fat; 1 g saturated fat; 1 g monounsaturated fat; 1 g polyunsaturated fat; 6 g carb; 1 g fiber; 2 g sugar; 55 mg calcium; 2 mg iron; 137 mg sodium; 402 mg potassium; 1148 IU vitamin A; 4 mg vitamin C; 127 mg cholesterol

Curried Chicken Meatball And Rice Skillet

Servings: 6

Ingredients:

- 1 slice Basic White Bread , made into crumbs
- 4 teaspoons curry powder, divided
- 1 large egg
- 1 tablespoon chopped fresh chives
- 1 pound ground chicken
- 2 tablespoons unsalted butter
- 1 tablespoon olive oil
- 1 medium onion, chopped
- 2 cloves garlic, minced
- 11/3 cups basmati rice
- 2 cups Chicken Stock
- 1/3 cup water
- 1/3 cup mango chutney
- 1 tablespoon lemon juice

Directions:

1. In medium bowl, combine bread crumbs, 2 teaspoons curry powder, egg, and chives and

mix well. Add ground chicken and mix gently to coat. Form into 16 meatballs.

2.   Combine unsalted butter and olive oil in a large saucepan over medium heat. When this mixture melts, add the meatballs and cook until browned, about 5 minutes, turning gently. Remove meatballs from skillet.

3.   Add onion and garlic to skillet; cook and stir to remove brown bits. Cook for another 5–6 minutes or until tender.

4.   Add rice and stir; cook for 1 minute longer. Add chicken stock, water, chutney, lemon juice, and remaining 2 teaspoons curry powder, and bring to a simmer.

5.   Return meatballs to skillet and cover; reduce heat to low. Simmer for 18–22 minutes or until rice is tender and the meatballs are done to 165°F. Serve immediately.

Nutrition Info: (Per Serving):Calories: 305; Total Fat: 9 g; Saturated Fat: 3 g; Cholesterol: 87 mg; Protein: 19 g; Sodium: 121 mg; Potassium: 158 mg; Fiber: 0 g; Carbohydrates: 33 g; Sugar: 1 g

Chicken In Orange Sauce

Servings: 4

Ingredients:

- 4 (6-ounce) boneless, skinless chicken breasts, cut into 1"-wide strips
- 1/8 teaspoon white pepper
- 3/4 cup orange juice, divided
- 2 tablespoons olive oil
- 1 tablespoon unsalted butter
- 1 tablespoon minced fresh ginger root
- 1 medium onion, finely chopped
- 1 teaspoon dried thyme leaves
- 2 tablespoons honey
- 2 tablespoons white wine vinegar
- 1 teaspoon grated orange zest
- 1/2 cup Chicken Stock
- 2 tablespoons cornstarch
- 2 tablespoons minced fresh chives

Directions:

1. Place chicken in bowl and sprinkle with white pepper and 2 tablespoons orange juice; toss to coat and set aside for 15 minutes.

2. Meanwhile, heat olive oil and butter in large saucepan over medium heat. Add ginger root and onion; cook and stir until tender, about 6–7 minutes.

3. In small bowl, combine remaining orange juice, thyme, honey, vinegar, orange zest, stock, and cornstarch and mix well; set aside.

4. Add chicken to skillet; cook, stirring frequently, until chicken is almost cooked through, about 5 minutes.

5. Stir orange-juice mixture and add to skillet. Cook, stirring constantly, until sauce thickens and bubbles and chicken is thoroughly cooked to 160°F. Sprinkle with chives and serve immediately.

Nutrition Info: (Per Serving):Calories: 288; Total Fat: 11 g; Saturated Fat: 3 g; Cholesterol: 73 mg; Protein: 27 g; Sodium: 86 mg; Potassium: 432 mg; Fiber: 0 g; Carbohydrates: 18 g; Sugar: 12 g

Java Chicken Paprika

Servings: 4

Ingredients:

- 1 pound boneless, skinless chicken breasts
- 1/2 cup fresh lemon juice
- 1/4 teaspoon freshly ground black pepper
- 1 tablespoon olive oil
- 1 large sweet onion, sliced
- 2 teaspoons paprika
- 1/2 teaspoon salt-free chili powder
- 1/2 teaspoon instant espresso powder
- 1/4 cup water
- 1 tablespoon cornstarch
- 1 tablespoon instant nonfat dry milk
- 1/2 cup skim milk
- Optional: Additional paprika, for garnish

Directions:

1. Place the chicken breasts between pieces of waxed paper or plastic wrap. Pound the breasts into thin pieces using a wooden mallet or rolling pin. Divide into 4 equal-sized pieces.
2. Place the chicken breasts in a small bowl. Pour the lemon juice over the chicken and

season with the freshly ground black pepper. Marinate for at least 5 minutes. Drain and pat dry, reserving the lemon juice.

3.   In a large nonstick skillet, heat the olive oil over medium heat. Add the onion and sauté until transparent, about 5–7 minutes. Remove the onion with a slotted spoon and set aside.

4.   Increase the heat to medium-high. Add the chicken breasts to the pan. Quick-fry the chicken breasts for about 1 minute on each side. Transfer the chicken to a serving platter and keep warm.

5.   Add the onion back to the pan and reheat. Add the paprika and chili powder; stir well. Add the espresso powder and water; bring to a boil.

6.   In a small bowl, whisk together the cornstarch, nonfat dry milk, and skim milk. Add the milk mixture and the reserved lemon juice to the pan; bring to a boil. Reduce heat and simmer, stirring until thickened.

7.   Spoon the sauce over the chicken. Sprinkle with additional paprika, if desired. Serve immediately.

Nutrition Info: (Per Serving):Calories: 214; Total Fat: 5 g; Saturated Fat: 0 g; Cholesterol: 66 mg; Protein: 28 g; Sodium: 111 mg; Potassium: 549 mg; Fiber: 1 g; Carbohydrates: 13 g; Sugar: 7 g

Lightning Source UK Ltd.
Milton Keynes UK
UKHW021101220721
387582UK00001B/43